I0440188

Healthy Lifestyle Report: Fitness

Proven Tips You Can Use

To

Get Fit and in Shape

RON KNESS

ISBN-13: 978-1535057769

ISBN-10: 1535057769

Contents

Introduction

We all know about certain benefits of exercising - above all, that it's good for us. But this isn't always enough to get us motivated into actually doing it. If you're looking for a little inspiration to get started, here are 10 reasons why exercise can improve your life.

1) **More Energy**: Although exercise in itself may be tiring, one of the major benefits of exercising is the fact that it'll ultimately leave you feeling more energized. Studies have shown that regular exercise helps to reduce fatigue.

2) **Increase Your Mood**: Every time you exercise your body will release endorphins that help to make you feel good. Exercise really will give you a natural high!

3) **Improve Your Health**: There are so many health benefits of losing weight that it's impossible to list them all here! By getting fit you'll reduce the risk of diabetes, cancer, high blood pressure, stroke, heart disease and much more.

4) **Improve Your Appearance**: If being overweight or not being toned leaves you feeling unhappy about yourself then losing weight can help you to look and feel better.

5) **Play With Your Kids**: It takes a lot of energy to keep up with your kids. By losing weight and getting fit, you'll be able to run around with them without constantly getting out of breath. This can be one of the most rewarding benefits of exercising: it helps you to enjoy life more.

6) **Sleep Better**: When you exercise more you'll start to find it easier to get a good night's rest. This adds to the energy boost that you'll get from exercise in the long term.

7) **Increase Your Strength and Stamina**: Do you find it hard to go on long walks, even though you want to? Or maybe even carrying shopping bags up the stairs is a struggle? Exercise more and you'll eventually be able to handle these activities with ease.

8) **Reduce Stress**: Exercise can hugely reduce stress levels. If you regularly suffer from stress - or even mental health issues such as depression and anxiety - regular exercise can help to reduce your symptoms.

9) **A Sense Of Achievement**: When you start to exercise and see the improvements you're making week on week, you'll really get the feeling that you've achieved something worthwhile!

10) **Keep Your Independence Later In Life**: The more you can exercise now, while you're still able, the more you can reduce the impact of certain health problems later in life. In short, keeping fit and healthy will help you to keep your independence as late into life as possible.

So how much will you need to work out to feel these benefits of exercising? That all depends on your current fitness levels. The good news is that just 30 minutes of exercise a day is enough to improve your health drastically. So what are you waiting for! Let's dig deeper into the world of fitness and how it can improve your life now and into the future.

The Benefits of Exercising

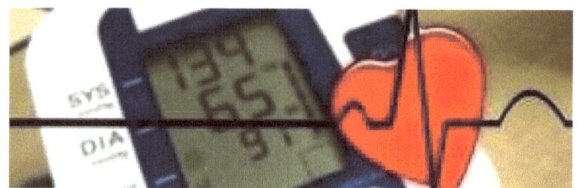

W hether you want to lose a few or a hundred pounds, it's crucial that you understand that the benefits of exercise go way beyond weight loss and cosmetic enhancement. Some benefits of exercise pertain to your health in particular.

Exercising often (3-4 times a week for 30 minutes to an hour each day) has been found by experts to greatly reduce the risk of several diseases and health conditions. Some diseases that exercise will help you prevent are heart disease, stroke, and Peripheral Vascular Disease.

High blood pressure and high cholesterol are both health conditions that could be avoided by regular exercise. Diabetes that's non-insulin-dependent can be controlled by eliminating body fat and increasing your daily physical activity.

Over 40% of American people alone are considered medically obese. This is caused by a lack of activity in their everyday life and the increase in fast food in their diets. By building muscle mass rather than fat, it will help your metabolism increase, which makes burning calories easier.

Most patients that come into a doctor's office complaining of back pain are overweight. Doing exercises that improve your flexibility, such as yoga, Pilates, and tai chi, for example will be able to help reduce back pain.

The benefits of exercise clearly go beyond weight loss. It's more than just making your body look great - it also makes your life-span increasingly longer so that you can enjoy your loved ones and all that life has to offer.

How Weight Training Benefits Your Heart

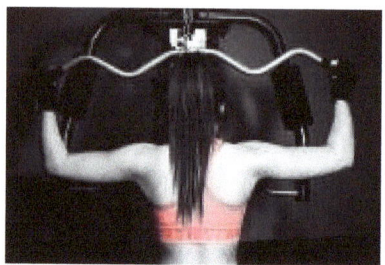

There's a lot of focus on aerobic activity for weight loss and improving the function of the heart. And there should be a lot of focus on it because it's very beneficial to heart health. However, weight training also has benefits for the heart that occur indirectly.

Weight training helps to increase the size of your skeletal muscles. When you increase the muscle tissue in your body, you naturally speed up your metabolism.

That's because muscle tissue burns a lot of energy in order to sustain itself. What that means for you is that you burn calories more efficiently.

And if you're trying to reduce the amount of body fat you have, having a strong underlying set of muscles is the fastest way to do that.

You can actually change your resting metabolism and burn more calories while you're at rest. That translates into more efficient weight loss.

This is important because having excess weight is a major risk factor when it comes to heart disease and stroke. By participating in an exercise program that includes weight training, you can actually help to improve your cardiac risk factors and reduce your chances of having a heart attack or other heart disease.

Weight training can also help to reduce your risk of diabetes because it helps the insulin in your blood to work properly.

The more sensitive your body is to insulin, the fewer problems you'll have with keeping your blood sugar levels stable. Diabetes is a major coronary risk factor; so keeping it at bay is heart healthy.

Weight training also helps to increase your physical strength as well as your bone density. That translates into an easier time performing exercises that are cardiovascular in nature.

When you have strong muscles and bones, you're better able to go for a brisk walk every day to get your heart pumping. You'll also have fewer injuries that prevent you from getting daily exercise.

In addition, strength training helps you to perform the tasks of daily life without as much difficulty.

For example, you'll be able to pick up your laundry basket more easily and take out the trash without straining. These may seem like small tasks, but for someone with heart disease they can be major.

Weight training should be moderate and guided by someone who knows how to help you best. People who have some serious heart complications may not be able to perform strength training safely.

Make sure to talk with your doctor about starting a physical fitness program that includes strength training.

Five Fun Exercises You Can Do Outdoors

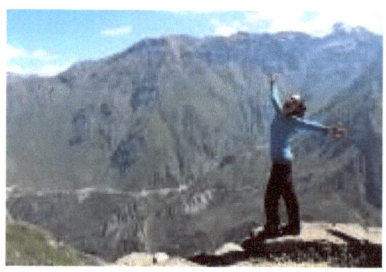

Want to know five fun exercises you can do outdoors? When you're outdoors, it makes it more fun to exercise since you can focus your mind on other things instead of how much your legs burn. Swimming is one of the top five fun exercises you can do outdoors.

Swimming works many aspects of your body: your lungs, legs, and arm muscles - not to mention it greatly strengthens the most important body part - your heart. Swimming allows you to get a great workout without having your body weigh you down with every move you make.

Hiking is also one of many fun exercises you do outdoors. There are many benefits of hiking - not just helping you control your body weight - but also improving your mental health as well. Pack a small, healthy lunch and set up a picnic once you reach a good resting spot.

Rock Climbing is another one of the top five fun exercises you can do outdoors. While you can do rock climbing inside, it's always better to get some fresh air. Rock climbing works mostly your arms and legs, but it also helps your lungs learn how to breathe better.

Biking is fun because you can do it basically anywhere, anytime! You can enjoy the scenery by yourself or you can bring a friend along. Just make sure you always wear your helmet for extra safety precautions while you get your workout in.

Obstacle courses are a great form of fun exercises. They work almost all aspects of your body and with each turn on the course, you can try to be faster. This will help you build endurance. These activities that you do outdoors will replace your fitness boredom with some healthy fun exercise activity!

On the Path Towards Health Fitness

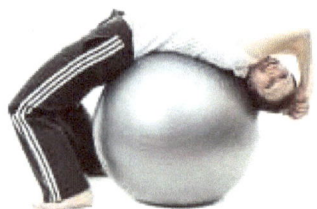

As far as being healthy is concerned, it clearly takes more than a well-sculpted physique or a radiant-looking skin to attest to your inner-self's well-being. A lot of people mistake being healthy as somewhat of a physical attribute. In reality, how we really take care of ourselves from the inside is what really counts. Health fitness is where we take care of ourselves from the inside, helping rid the body off viruses and bacteria that may cause us to get sick or have infections. Maintaining proper health fitness requires us to really go all-natural to stay fit and healthy.

Here are a few simple tips to help you get on track towards health fitness:

Get Busy - In today's busy, busy world, an "active lifestyle" is often misconstrued as having tons of work, going from errand to errand, but in reality, such a lifestyle can only cause our health fitness more damage than good. What I actually mean by getting busy is to make the most of our body, give it a little "exercise" whenever we can.

Not all of us have the time (nor the money) for the gym, so taking the stairs instead of the elevator when going to work is a healthy and effective alternative. Also, when doing errands, try as much as possible to not use the car especially if it's not that far. You not only save gas but you give yourself muscles a healthy boost.

Moving around and making the most of what your body can do for you (without overdoing it of course!) doesn't only keep you in shape, your health fitness at good levels but it also keeps you in a better mood.

Stress Busters - Speaking of keeping yourself in a good mood, there's this common misconception that whenever you feel frustrated or angry, releasing and lashing out those pent up emotions are actually good for your health. Sounds familiar? Well, studies show that this is just a myth. People who have pent up anger and release it through hostile means only makes them more prone to strokes and heart attacks.

Apparently, instead of helping you "release" those bad vibes, it actually just makes you more hostile and angry, thus, possibly resulting to a stroke, heart disease, high-blood pressure and the like. To help you stay cool and your health fitness well, try to stay calm whenever faced with stress or anything that angers you.

Avoiding anger or stressful situations is really the best way to keep your health fitness at its best.

Change Your Exercise Mindset and Change Your Life (and Body)

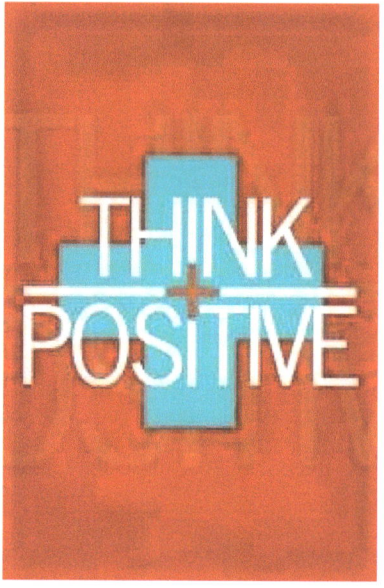

Exercise is fun, right? Well it's not fun for everyone. In fact, many people consider it nothing short of torture. Perhaps it's because they've fallen prey to many of the myths about exercise. Changing your exercise mindset, and letting go of these myths, can change your life.

No Pain No Gain

How often have you heard this lovely cliché? It implies that exercise must be painful in order for it to work. That's just not true. Believing it is a sure-fire way to avoid exercise too! Who wants to feel intense pain? Actually, exercise can and should be fun and something you can do each and every day. Because honestly - if you're not having fun, how likely are you to continue doing it?

If it's not easy to do, how can you find time to fit it into your day?

It's a whole lot easier to motivate yourself to go for a walk or a bike ride to the store than it is to run five miles, right? And you can fit a walk into your day every day. It's easier to go play tennis with a friend than to climb on the stair machine at the local gym. And much more fun, too.

You Have to Exercise to Be Healthy

More and more, scientists and doctors are learning that movement is more important than exercise. Exercise tends to be defined as sustained activity for twenty, thirty, or even sixty minutes. It's a spin class, the time it takes to run three miles or an hour on the treadmill. However, studies are showing that it's more beneficial to have a practice of moving your body rather than "exercising."

Moving your body means walking; it means being physically active. It doesn't mean an hour in the spin class – unless you enjoy spin class. Exercise is fine as long as it's part of a daily habit of movement. Instead of sitting at your desk for four hours, getting lunch and returning to your desk, get up and take a five-minute walk each hour. If you can, stand at your desk. Bike to work. Walk to the coffee shop or store.

Adopting a Healthy, and Active, Mindset

If you dread working out, find an activity that you enjoy. The activity should require movement – knitting or watching Dancing with the Stars doesn't count. However dancing, playing tennis, hiking, playing golf, swimming are all great activities. Do something you enjoy that gets your body moving.

Additionally, take a look at your current habits. What can you replace with movement?

Where can you fit physical activity into your day? It doesn't have to be a five mile run; it can be a one mile walk. The important thing is to move.

 If you like goals and numbers, shoot for ten thousand steps a day. That's about five miles and to reach that number each day, you'll likely have to create a few new habits (and lose a few old ones). You can do it. Your health depends on it. To your success!

Strength Training Basics

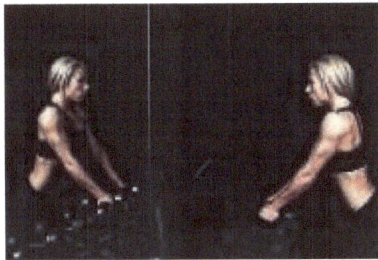

M any people want to start a strength training program but aren't sure how to do so, or what to do. If you are completely new to strength training, you will want to start out easy. Never push yourself until you've done this awhile and know when and how you can push yourself.

It should be noted that the terms strength training, weight training and resistance training can be used synonymously. It's generally a person preference as to the terminology people use.

Before we get into the basics of strength training, let's discuss some of the benefits.

This type of training will help you increase your strength, giving you more physical power, which can help you get through your daily tasks easier and allow you to have more endurance to do things like yard work, hiking, playing with your kids and many other things.

Getting your muscles toned and in shape with strength training will also improve your balance and coordination. It helps increase your balance because you work opposing muscle groups. For example, if your abdominal muscles are strong, but your back muscles are weak, this can affect how well you balance your body, even while standing erect.

It can also lead to injury of your back because those muscles are weak.

Working out with strength training can also help you decrease your body fat and lower your risk of certain diseases associated with being overweight. Diseases like diabetes and high blood pressure are related to your weight and overall health putting you at a higher risk of having these problems.

The basics:

Repetitions

Strength training consists of doing sets and reps (or repetitions.) A repetition is the full range of motion you put each muscle group through. A full rep is made up of an eccentric contraction and a concentric contraction. The eccentric contraction of the muscle, which lengthens it and the concentric contraction of the muscle, which shortens it.

For example, with a bicep curl, when your arms are stretched out (or hanging) by your sides this is the eccentric part of the repetition. When you raise the weight so your elbows are bent and your hands are close to your shoulders, this is the concentric portion of the rep.

Some people refer to this at the bottom and top of a rep too. The bottom is the eccentric part, while the concentric part is the top of a rep.

Sets

A set is made up of a number of repetitions. If you decide to do 12 repetitions of bicep curls, that is considered one set. You can do however many of reps you want, whether it's 8, 10, 12, etc. You have to judge how many reps you can do in proper form.

For example, if you do 8 reps of 3 sets, that is actually 24 times you will go through the motion of lifting the weight. However, you should rest in between sets, but not between reps. You know when you have done enough of if you are lifting the right amount of weight when your muscles cannot do another repetition when you are at the end of your set.

Use proper form to avoid injury

You want to do each rep properly and slowly. If you get sloppy this can indicate that you are trying to lift too much weight or do too many reps at that weight. You will need to adjust either the weight you are lifting or the number of reps you are performing for each set. You want to be in control of the weight. Do not let it dangle or flail around. Doing so can lead to injury and will actually stop you from gaining the benefits of weight lifting.

Results

It's likely you will not see visible results for a while. This can be due to the fact that you may have too much body fat and it will need to be decreased before you see the muscle tone underneath. It will also depend on how responsive your muscles are to weight training. Some people can build or tone muscles very quickly, while for others it takes a lot of time and work. Do not get discouraged if you don't see fast results. The benefits in strength and endurance far outweigh how good you look in a tee-shirt.

Goals

Depending on the goals you're trying to reach, you will want to devise a strength training plan that fits your needs. If you're simply wanting to increase your endurance, but not necessarily build muscle, you will use light weights and work on adding more reps per set.

If you want to increase your strength or build muscle, you will use moderate to heavy weights and do fewer reps per set.

Examples:

For endurance you may use a 5 pound dumbbell for bicep curls and do 15 reps for each set. You may gradually increase this to 20 or 25 reps per set.

Eventually you will need to add some weight, maybe move up to a 7 pound dumbbell and back off your reps to 15 again and work up to 20 or 25.

Always remember that any time you increase the weight you are lifting, you need to decrease the reps per set and work your way back up again.

For strength and building muscle you may start with a 10, 15 or 20 pound dumbbell for bicep curls and only do 8 reps per set. You will gradually work up to 10 sets and then 12. At that time you need to increase the weight of your dumbbell and drop your reps back down to 8 again.

This is just the very basics of strength training and terminology. If you want to simply build endurance, have better muscle tone and decrease your risk of weight related diseases, then it's likely a simple home workout with a few dumbbells is plenty for you.

If you want to go hard core into weight training or body building, it's best to join a gym and seek the advice of a personal trainer.

Whatever your goals, always strive to use proper form and never do more than you handle. An injury can put you back for weeks. If you need to see proper techniques, you can visit YouTube and find videos uploaded by professionals that will get you started on the right track.

Improve Your Cardio

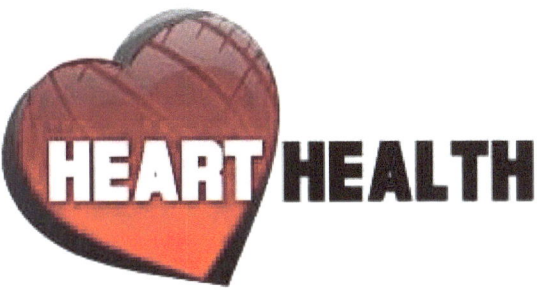

I f you are looking to trim down and tone up for the summer, you really need to be incorporating cardiovascular exercise into your routine.

Why Is Cardio Important?

Cardiovascular workouts get your heart rate working, the blood pumping, and the pounds falling off. It is one of the most important components of a well-rounded exercise regimen.

What Can Cardio Do for Me?

A great cardio workout can help you shed pounds and target problem areas, not to mention how important it is for heart and overall health.

How Much Cardio Should I Be Doing?

It is recommended that you get at least 30 minutes of cardiovascular exercise per day or more. You can, however, combine that amount into specific days' workouts. For example, you can do one hour of cardio every other day.

I Don't Have Time to Go to a Gym; Can I Get Enough Cardio in My Own Home?

Absolutely; there are tons of cardio workouts that you can do from home. Most require little to no equipment, and you can also get home workout machines to help you.

Home Cardio Exercises

* *Jump Rope* - You can purchase a jump rope very inexpensively at most sporting or department stores. This simple piece of equipment is one of the very best cardiovascular workouts and can actually be a lot of fun. You remember how to do it from when you were a kid, and you will be surprised how much it gets your heart rate up.

* *Trampoline* - Whether you go outside and use your kids' giant trampoline, or purchase a small single use trampoline for your home, simply bouncing around on one of these is a great cardio workout. You can do it while you are watching television or listening to music, and it is fun to work in lots of arm and hip movements as well.

* *Walking/Jogging* - Using a treadmill, your staircase, or getting outside for a walk or jog is perhaps the easiest way for anyone to get some great cardiovascular exercise. A brisk walk around your neighborhood can do wonders for your overall health and fitness level.

* *Aerobic Exercises* - These days, you can download, purchase, or watch exercise videos of all types just about anywhere. Aerobics, Jazzercise, Zumba and more are all excellent cardio workouts that you can do in the comfort of your own home.

* ***Home Machinery*** - If you have the room and budget for it, you can purchase gym equipment for your own home. Machines like treadmills, elliptical machines and stationary bikes are excellent for getting regular cardiovascular exercise.

Cardio workouts are more than just great workouts for weight loss and shedding pounds for bathing suit season. Getting enough cardio is important for your overall health and is one of the most important parts of a heart-healthy lifestyle.

You can improve your cardio by working these simple exercises into your daily life, or increasing your cardio workouts to something a little more intensive if your heart rate isn't quite high enough. On top of it all, cardio workouts are guaranteed to make you feel great as well as look great.

Why We Get Stiches When Running and How to Avoid Them

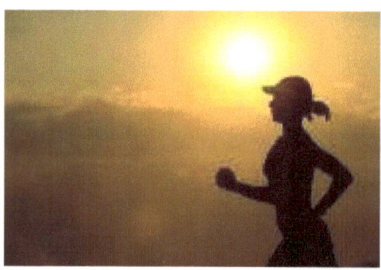

S ide stitches, or side pains, can be very painful and uncomfortable, and can hinder a perfect running experience almost immediately. The pain can start off slight and increase sharply in a matter of seconds. More than anything, side stitches are a nuisance to runners and may mean you need to stop your workout early!

What is a Stitch?

A side stitch is felt on either the right or left hand side of the body, though it most often occurs on the left side. It resonates in the area right below your lower ribs. The pain can be so intense at times that it can even cause you to stop running completely.

Why do Stitches Occur?

There is no definite medical explanation for why stitches occur, especially during running, but there are several theories. Some researchers claim that stitches are more common with beginner runners, due to the fact that they are more likely to engage in rapid or shallow breathing.

Rapid breathing is believed to not fully engage and relax the diaphragm, thereby causing the ligaments on one side of the body to contract forcefully. Another belief is that the rapid breathing, combined with the jolting of running and exhaling as your right foot touches the ground, puts additional strain on the ligaments near the liver and the diaphragm, which then causes the pain to be felt on the left side of the body.

Other research states that eating a meal within one hour of a run can cause side stitches, as well as drinking sugary or carbonated drinks. The digestive system has not worked the food and drinks completely through the system, and could be the reason for the sharp pains felt on the side.

Still other research suggests that if a runner forgoes a proper warm-up before a running session, and starts off running too fast, too soon, he or she will experience sharp side pain.

Preventing Stitches

If you notice that you get side stitches often, first ensure that you are not eating any type of meal, even a small snack, and large amounts of liquid within one to two hours of a run. You can drink a little water, but not too much, and avoid sports and carbonated drinks. Water is always your best choice before a run, especially in hot weather.

Another means of preventing stitches is to practice deep breathing in a rhythmic manner. Smooth, slow, complete breathing cycles will allow you to avoid rapid breathing. While you are breathing in and out fully, you also want to maintain proper posture.

The proper posture for running is to have your back straight, not hunched over, your chest up and open for easy breathing, and your arms bent at 90 degree angles at your sides.

This posture will ensure that your muscles are not being squeezed, which can cause almost a muscle cramp.

If you do happen to experience stitches, press real hard into the side that hurts and breathe deeply. Although it is hard to keep a good posture during this episode, try your best. After slow, even-paced breathing and massaging of the tense muscle, the pain should subside.

Stretching Should Be Part of Your Daily Routine

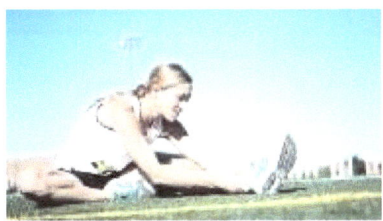

S tretching should be an integral part of your daily routine. It's something you should do several times a day. If you pay attention to dogs, cats and other animals, they always stretch when they get up from laying down. As you know, they don't have near the health problems or joint problems that humans do.

Stretching is a very important part of your fitness routine and can make the difference between a successful workout and one that doesn't bring you the results you need. Lack of stretching can even lead to injuries.

Here is some important information you should know about stretching.

Stretching is essential to your health and your mobility. It can also help you make progress faster than if you don't stretch before, during and after workouts. Stretching before your workout will help prepare the muscles for the workout that follows by loosening them up and getting them warmed up. This can help prevent injuries like tears in the ligaments, muscle strains and bone fractures.

Stretching also helps increase blood flow in your body and gets oxygen to all of your internal organs and tissues.

Benefits of Stretching:

- Improves muscle tone

- Helps reduce muscle stiffness and cramping

- Adds more flexibility

- Can help ease back pain

You should always include stretching as a regular part of your workout to help improve your posture, build stronger muscles and help improve your circulation. Not only that it's great for relieving stress and tension and helps you manage your overall stress levels and improves mental clarity. This is why yoga is so popular.

Always stretch before starting any exercise as a warm up, and then again after you exercise as a cool down. If you're running short on time and think you can skip stretching, you'd be better off to do the stretches and skip the workout. It doesn't matter whether you're into strength training or doing aerobic activity, you will benefit from warming up with a stretching routine.

A good way to get warmed up is to walk in place for a few minutes so your muscles start to warm up and you get some blood pumping. After that, spend five to ten minutes doing some stretches to further prepare your muscles for the workout ahead. Stretching cold muscles isn't good for them, so be sure to do some type of warm-up first.

However, this doesn't mean you can't stretch when you stand up after sitting for a while. Just be gentle and do light stretches. You want to do fuller and deeper stretches for your workouts, but a nice gentle stretch is great after long periods of sitting.

When stretching for a workout, you want to go into a stretch as far as you feel comfortable. Don't overdo it. You muscles will feel a little tight. After a minute or two they should start to feel more relaxed. You should be able to feel them release the tension.

Your cool down routine should include more stretching. This helps to relax the muscles and lengthen them to help you avoid cramps and injury. It's also good for your joints by having the muscles pull on the ligaments and tendons. This helps to keep them in good shape too. The last 10 minutes of your exercise routine should be dedicated to stretching.

Stretching is a vital part of a fitness routine. All top and professional athletes incorporate stretching into their daily workout. By including it as part of your regular workout, you will soon notice how beneficial it is. You will improve your exercise routine and you will feel better, move better, and think more clearly.

Start stretching as much as you can. It's the perfect way to start and end all of your workout sessions.

Elliptical vs Treadmill – How Do They Compare?

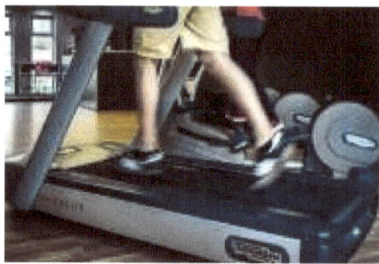

If you are a fitness enthusiast it won't be long before you start thinking of buying a home fitness machine. The two most popular exercise equipment for the home are the treadmill and elliptical trainer. Read on for a comparison of an elliptical vs treadmill. Which one is best for you?

Treadmill

A treadmill is an exercise machine that allows you to jog, walk or run while staying in one place. It can even simulate walking up a small hill. Many treadmill models today have preset programs and intensity levels to choose from. This allows you to choose a workout that will match your fitness goal.

Elliptical Trainer

Elliptical trainers are a relatively new addition to the line of fitness machines, but they are rapidly gaining popularity. Elliptical trainers provide a low impact exercise that can be compared to running in mid-air. They work out both the lower and upper body.

Compare Elliptical vs Treadmill

Walking and running are popular forms of exercise. That's because these are two activities that practically everybody can do.

Walking or running outdoors is great, but there are times when it's not practical. For instance, you wouldn't want to go out in the rain or snow. If you want to exercise anytime you feel like it, you will want to have your own home fitness machine.

The question is, should you buy an elliptical trainer or a treadmill? Let's compare elliptical vs treadmill so you can decide for yourself.

Calories burned. A treadmill provides an excellent lower body workout for the legs, thighs and buttocks. An elliptical works out both the lower and upper body. You may think an elliptical trainer burns more calories than a treadmill but the difference is really not that much. If you want to burn more calories, exercise harder and longer!

Possibility of injury. An elliptical provides low-impact exercise and is recommended for people with joint or back problems. Treadmills can have a higher incidence of injury for the simple reason that running on a treadmill is a high impact activity. This is not to say that nobody can suffer an injury on an elliptical. To reduce your chance of injury, warm up properly and build up the intensity of your workout gradually.

Cost. The cost of treadmills and ellipticals can range from a few hundred to a few thousand dollars, depending on the quality and features. On average, ellipticals are more affordable than treadmills.

Durability. Comparing elliptical vs treadmill, an elliptical trainer is more durable because it has fewer moving parts.

Space requirements. Quality treadmills and ellipticals require a sizeable amount of space. However, there are treadmills that you can fold up and store when not in use.

Ellipticals require floor space dedicated for its use.

Elliptical vs Treadmill: The Verdict

An elliptical trainer offers a total body workout and provides a low impact exercise. In this sense it excels over the treadmill. However, personal preferences always come into play and you may find that a treadmill works best for you. As to whether you should get an elliptical vs treadmill, the final decision is yours. Just remember to consult a health professional before you start any exercise program.

Strength Training Burns Fat

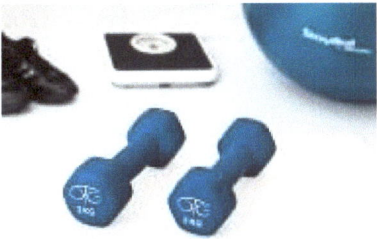

W hile the best way to burn fat is through aerobic exercise, you can also burn fat with certain types of strength training. The reason is that the more muscle you have, the more fat you can burn though normal activities. You can also combine aerobic exercise with strength training to get a double whammy effect against fat.

Don't Worry about Bulking Up

Strength training doesn't necessarily have to bulk you up. It can actually tone your body and help build your muscles just enough to help hold your body in more perfect alignment. Doing so can help you appear thinner and reduce body fat at the same time.

Try Circuit Training

This is something you can find at different studios that involve doing each machine for a specific period of time - usually at a fast pace. It's a good way to get both cardio in and strength training. Usually there is little or no rest in between each machine and exercise are done in between machines.

Isometric Weight Training

This is a type of resistance training where you use the weights by holding them at certain angles for 30 seconds to one minute instead of doing faster repetitions. This kind of strength training can also be done without weights. For instance, doing planks works well too. It increases strength and stamina.

High Volume Training

This type of strength training involves working one muscle group per week, concentrating on cardiovascular the rest of the time. This gives the muscle groups ample time to recover allowing for the best and most efficient building of strength training without bulking up your muscles. You can have long, lean muscles with high volume training.

Core Exercises

Doing core strength training exercises such as Pilates and yoga will help your body become a fat burning furnace. Try hot yoga, or purchase a Pilates machine to use at home for no excuse workouts that build endurance while building strength. The better shape your core is in, the better your fitness level will be and the more fat you'll burn.

Using your own body, bands or other methods to provide resistance during exercise will build your strength and muscles which will also burn more fat off your body. The great thing about resistance training is that you can combine it with cardio for increased results. Using simple tools such as bands, or workout equipment like the resistance exercise chair.

Mixed Exercise: Cardio Plus Strength Training Combined

Many exercise gurus have put out videos and programs that combine cardio with resistance training that work extra well. You can typically work out for half the time by combining the two together in creative ways and burn more calories. You can seriously blast fat away with these programs.

Cardio Then Strength Training

You can also burn fat by doing the exercises separately. The strength training builds muscle, which burns more fat, and the cardio burns fat. You can do the cardio and the strength training together or separately. Studies show that it doesn't really matter, other than the fact that when you do it together you can do it in half the time.

Burning fat through strength training is a two-pronged effort. You'll need to combine strength training with some sort of cardiovascular exercise for it to be the most effective and to avoid having bulky muscles. But, for long-term fitness goals, this is your fat burning answer.

Setting Realistic Fitness Goals

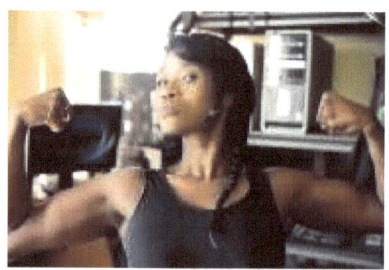

H ow often have you decided to start getting fit and add more exercise to your daily routine? How often have you given up before you even start? I know, you want to set really good fitness goals. You have good intentions, but you give up too soon. This is often from setting unrealistic goals for yourself. If you decide you're going to start walking three miles a day, in the beginning that's probably unrealistic, especially if you don't currently engage in anything physical. A better goal is to aim for one mile per day and work your way up to three or more. Give yourself plenty of time for the goal.

If you decide that you're going to reach the three mile goal in one month, you need to keep evaluating how you're doing each week and readjust your goal to a later date if needed. Don't give up, just modify your goals.

Do things you enjoy. If you don't enjoy a daily walk, it's likely you won't stick to it. Instead you can try kickboxing, Zumba dance, aerobics, swimming, or anything you'll have fun doing. There's also martial arts if you're in the mood for a little discipline. Whatever you choose, it needs to be fun, interesting and something you can modify or change up routines if you need to.

Start easy. If you've been laying around and not doing anything, you need to start in very small increments. If five minutes is all you can handle, then start there. Maybe you can do five minutes a few times per day. Instead of setting a starting goal of thirty minutes per day, break it up throughout the day. You don't have to do the whole thirty minutes at one time. In fact, if you start in five to ten minute increments you will probably enjoy it more plus you'll start seeing progress within a week or two.

Keep yourself motivated. Listen to upbeat music, read daily affirmations, meditate. Do whatever it takes to keep yourself motivated. Many people stop exercise programs because they lose motivation or have no one to motivate them. Tell yourself that you're going to work on daily motivation no matter if other people support you or not. Your health is about you, it's not about them.

Celebrate successes. Whenever you reach a milestone or fitness goal, be sure to reward yourself. However, instead of rewarding yourself with a sweet treat you might want to consider something you'll use or something you want. It can be a new mp3 player, a new shirt, or a new pair of jeans.

Use a calendar or notebook. You need some kind of journal to judge your progress. Using a daily journal will help keep you on track and let you know if you need to make adjustments to your current program.

Getting into shape and improving your health will take time. Set realistic goals and keep records of your progress. As you reach milestones in your level of fitness you'll find new motivation to keep going. Remember to start small and work your way up.

Conclusion

As you can see, exercising is important for a number of reasons. Not only does it help you manage your weight, but builds muscle mass which increases the speed of your metabolism, thus burning more calories – even while you sleep.

As we age, the body tends to get more fragile. Not only do we lose muscle, but we lose flexibility and balance. These can lead to falls and breakage of bones of which many seniors never fully recover.

Regular exercise helps preserve balance and flexibility by not only reducing your risk of falling, but by making normal everyday tasks easier. Range of motion and increased muscle mass allows you to maintain your independence well into your Golden Years.

Don't let a lack of initiative now affect you later. Try to get at least some exercise most days. An ideal program would be 30 minutes of cardio four days per week, 30 minutes of strength training two days per week (but not on consecutive days) and resting on the seventh day.

Add to that a sensible healthy eating plan to manage your weight and your senior years should be some of the best years of your life.

Other Health Reports By This Author

If you would like to read more health reports on various topics, here is a list of CreateSpace titles and descriptions:

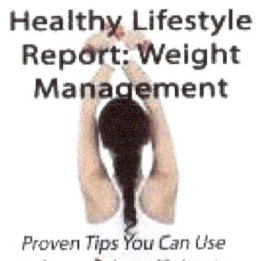

Nutrition

Nutrition is at the heart of losing weight and good health. In fact 80% of weight loss has to do with eating healthy with the other 20% about exercise. Good nutrition starts with three areas:

- What you eat

- How much you eat

- When you eat.

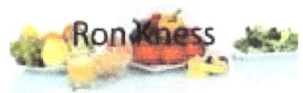

Weight Management

Losing weight in theory is easy. All you have to do is burn more calories than what you eat. If your deficit is 3,500 calories in a week, you'll lose one pound.

The problem is there are many more factors at play that can affect weight loss than just calories, such as emotions, stress, illness, hormones, menstruation, etc. So it is not easy, but with a healthy lifestyle program it is doable.

Fat Burning/Motivational Tips

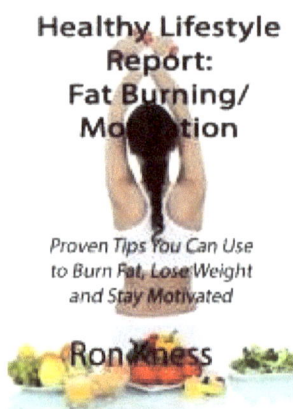

Be honest: When you look in a mirror, which bit do you hate the most? Is it those 'Love Handles' that have sprouted up?

This excess fat goes on so easy, so why does it require so much effort to make it come off again? Is it possible to burn more fat? Yes it is and we show you how in this report , along with giving you some motivation to keep going on your weight loss journey.

Senior Health

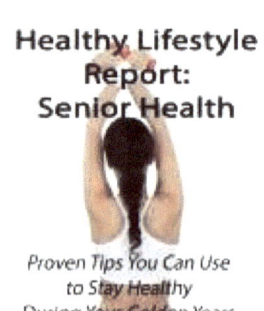

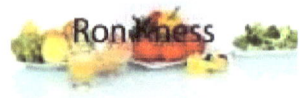

Retirement should be one of the best times of your life, but health issues caused by being overweight can not only limit your mobility, but cause a whole host of health problems. In this report, we discuss how to eat right, exercise and deal with some of the issues of aging.

Be sure to check back at CreateSpace at *https://www.createspace.com* frequently for new health reports. Just go to the Store and Search for "Ron Kness" (without the quotes of course) for a list of my books and reports.

About the Author

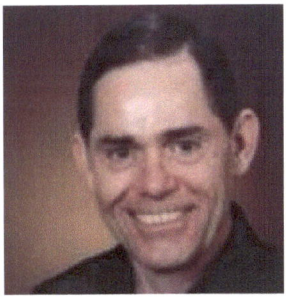 I grew up in Central Minnesota, where my parents owned and operated a fishing resort. Once out of high school I tried a couple of semesters of college, only to quit halfway through the Spring term; I decided at that time that college wasn't for me.

Then I decided to follow my father's previous occupation as an auto mechanic. I graduated from a two-year of vocational training course and worked as a mechanic. While in vocational training, I decided to join the National Guard where I eventually ended up working full-time for 32 years.

So how does all of this relate to writing? In one of my leadership schools, the instructor, who was an English teacher at a juvenile detention center, presented writing to me in a whole new way - a way that started to develop my interest in working with words.

Fast forward about 40 years and I now have over 50 books listed on Amazon for Kindle and CreateSpace.

Besides my own writing, I also ghostwrite ebooks, reports, articles, blogs and do Kindle conversions for my clients on a variety of topics.

Today my wife and I live in Gold Canyon, AZ, where you'll find me happily sitting in my office typing away on my laptop as I work on my next book or ghostwriting project . . . that is if we are not traveling on a cruise ship - our new-found mode of travel.

www.ingramcontent.com/pod-product-compliance
Lightning Source LLC
Chambersburg PA
CBHW050845290526
45792CB00002B/526